THE COMPLETE USAGE GUIDE: CLOBETASOL PROPIONATE

The essential guide on everything you need to know about clobetasol propionate to aid with eczema and psoriasis

DR. LEWIS FREEMAN

Contents

CHAPTER ONE 4
Understanding Clobetasol propionate 4
Modes of Administration 8
Benefits of Clobetasol propionate 14
Potential Side Effects 20
Alternatives 22
CHAPTER TWO 24
Interactions with other medications 24
When to seek medical attention 26
Safety Precautions and mistakes to avoid while using clobetasol propionate 29
Duration of treatment and when to stop 32
THE END 38

CHAPTER ONE

Understanding Clobetasol propionate

Clobetasol propionate is a skin applied medication that helps to treat a variety of skin problems such as itching, burning, swelling, reddening, along with other sensitive skin disorders such as eczema, psoriasis, lichen planus, and dermatitis. And it does this by hindering the immune response processes which results to a reduction of inflammation in the affected areas. Clobetasol propionate is an effective solution for all kinds of skin disorders and the good thing is that it comes in different forms to suit its different modes of administration on the different affected areas of the skin. However effective this medication may prove to be in treating skin problems, it's important to always consult your dermatologist before and during usage in order to better understand the potential side effects, the dosage instruction and administration. Seek the help of your skincare professional if you experience any skin reactions upon usage of clobetasol propionate.

Modes of Administration

The most popular mode of application of clobetasol propionate is by direct application or administration of the cream or ointment on the surface affected area of the skin. This is done by gently massaging the cream or ointment on the affected layer of the skin. Always avoid rigorous rubbing as it could lead to further unwanted skin complications. Also, excess use of the cream or ointment could result to inflammation which would in-turn birth skin itching, reddening, swelling, irritations, as well as other skin disorders.

When the affected area of the skin is the scalp, the best form of clobetasol propionate to use for the affected area is clobetasol. This is done by rubbing the clobetasol on the scalp and massaging thoroughly in order to have the affected area of the scalp treated. Clobetasol is best used to treating dandruff and reducing inflammation. In case of dermatitis, and scaling; use clobetasol shampoo to massage the scalp thoroughly. This process when properly done reduces scaling and puts dandruff, dermatitis and psoriasis to bed for good.

The best form of clobetasol propionate for treating affected hairy regions of the skin is the clobetasol foam. This is used by direct application onto the hairy regions of the affected skin. Frequently applying clobetasol foam into the affected hairy areas would go a long way in treating scaling, psoriasis, and dandruff; hence bring about relief in the infected skin layers.

Benefits of Clobetasol propionate

Due to its powerful and effective nature, clobetasol propionate has proven to have numerous advantages especially in the area of ensuring a health, problem-free skin.

Clobetasol propionate is solely responsible for hindering the immune response system, thereby reducing skin inflammation, and treating skin reactions such as swelling, reddening, itching, irritations, and burning. It's also responsible for treating skin disorders such as psoriasis, lichen planus, skin discoloration, eczema, and dermatitis; amongst other serious skin disorders.

Another reason to consider clobetasol propionate is in its distinct varieties specially made for its administration on the different areas of the skin. For infections on the surface level of the skin; clobetasol creams and ointments are best applied for rapid effectivess. For issues around hairy regions, clobetasol foams are best applied for maximum results. Another form of clobetasol propionate is the clobetasol shampoo applied on scalp affected areas in order to treat scaling, dandruff and inflammation.

Clobetasol propionate has rapid response rate of effectiveness. A thorough application of the medication brings instant relief and comfort to the infected area of the skin. It is also effective in treating a host of skin conditions such as eczema, psoriasis, dermatitis, lichen planus, and other skin disorders that are susceptible to other skincare medications.

As long as the dosage prescriptions and instructions of a doctor or dermatologist are followed, the chances of after-use skin reactions or irritations are minimal.

Potential Side Effects

Although effective, when excessively or inappropriately used or abused could result to inflammation and a host of unwanted skin reactions and disorders such as skin discoloration, swelling, scaling, burning, eczema, dermatitis, lichen planus, itching, reddening, and stretch marks along with other skin disorders.

Always consult your dermatologist or skincare

professional for proper guidance before and during the usage of this medication. Report any skin reaction to your dermatologist.

Alternatives

Despite the variety and number of alternatives for clobetasol creams, it is advisable to seek the counsel of your skincare professional in order to be sure which alternative cream would best serve your condition.

CHAPTER TWO

Interactions with other medications

Clobetasol propionate can interact with a host of other medications such as vitamins, drugs or herbs; resulting in its ineffectiveness. Hence, endeavor to talk to your doctor or medical guardian about all the medications you are currently taking before embarking on clobetasol propionate. Your healthcare guardian will be best placed to ascertain what drugs, vitamins or herbs are safe to take along with clobetasol propionate, and the ones which are to be avoided.

When to seek medical attention

The importance of seeking the guidance of a skincare professional cannot be overemphasized. Diligently adhering to the instructions given by your doctor or dermatologist would go a long way in helping you avoid unwanted skin reactions and irritations. Do not hesitate to report to your skincare guardian when you experience skin reactions such as reddening, swelling, itching, scaling, skin discoloration; as well as other skin disorders such as eczema, psoriasis, dermatitis and lichen planus. Seek medical attention before combining this medication with other drugs, vitamins or herbs of any nature to avoid an interaction of the drugs and hence ineffectiveness.

Safety Precautions and mistakes to avoid while using clobetasol propionate

In order to achieve maximum result certain precautions should be taken and errors should be avoided while using this medication. Excessive use of this medication leads to increased inflammation which gives room to itching, irritation, swelling, burning and skin discoloration. Always avoid an excessive use of this medication especially on the affected area. Frequently rubbing the cream or ointment on the same affected area or region would lead to further complications. Also avoid applying this cream on physical injuries, and it could end up elongating the healing process of the injuries. Avoid using this medication on sensitive areas of the body as it could result in injuries, reddening, irritations, or swelling of such sensitive areas.

Duration of treatment and when to stop

The duration of treatment depends largely on the level of damage done to the affected area of the skin, and when to cease treatment is very much dependent on the effective response of the medication in treating skin problems. It's important to stop using the skincare medication only when skin disorders such as irritations, swelling, itching, eczema, etc. are completely neutralized. The general duration for the use of this skincare medication is about 3-4 weeks. It is best to seek the guidance of your doctor or skincare professional, and endeavor to adhere to his instructions as he would help you minimize the chances of a side effect; thereby maximizing the effectiveness of clobetasol propionate.

THE END

www.ingramcontent.com/pod-product-compliance
Lightning Source LLC
Chambersburg PA
CBHW072049230526
45479CB00009B/331